3 books in 1

I0441690

Copyright © 2016 HTeBooks

Disclaimer

This book is designed to provide condensed information. It is not intended to reprint all the information that is otherwise available, but instead to complement, amplify and supplement other texts. You are urged to read all the available material, learn as much as possible and tailor the information to your individual needs.

Every effort has been made to make this book as complete and as accurate as possible. However, there may be mistakes, both typographical and in content. Therefore, this text should be used only as a general guide and not as the ultimate source of information. The purpose of this book is to educate.

The author or the publisher shall have neither liability nor responsibility to any person or entity regarding any loss or damage caused, or alleged to have been caused, directly or indirectly, by the information contained in this book.

Table of Contents

How To Drink Tea for Weight Loss

People have been looking for all kinds of ways to cut their weight down. Some tried all kinds of exercise and diet programs. Others tried consuming various foods and concoctions in the hope of removing extra inches and pounds fast. Others go for extreme measures, even if these entail high cost and the potential of life-threatening side effects. However, only a few people know that what they need to lose weight has always been there for centuries.

This is mainly the objective of this book: "How to Drink Tea for Weight Loss: Healthy Tea Recipes That Will Help You Lose Weight Fast". The main aim of this book is to educate people of the natural wonders of drinking tea and the ways it can help people to lose weight. This book aims to educate people about the unique weight-shaving abilities of tea, as well as its other health-giving properties. It will also show people how to prepare tea the right way so they can lose weight in the most efficient way.

The contents of this book, in no particular order, are as follows.

1. The health properties of tea - Tea is one of the first drinks humans discovered. While it is popular as a drink fit for social gatherings, the main reason for it sticking to the consciousness of communities everywhere is that it helps in improving one's well-being. From how it helps with digestion to how its chemical components stimulate the body to run more efficiently, this book will take a more detailed look on the health properties of tea.

2. The different kinds of tea - Drinking tea in general is always good for you. Of course, not all teas are equal. There are numerous variations of tea available on the market and each of them has different properties. Learning about their different traits would help you appreciate your tea better while improving your knowledge on how tea helps your body.

3. How to prepare tea the right way-True, tea enthusiasts know that the way you prepare tea has a huge say on the quality of the final product. If you do not know how to prepare tea correctly, then you will not get the quality you desire. This book will guide you on how you can prepare tea like a pro and get a high quality result. Not only will you get great-tasting tea this way, but it will also help in getting the most out of the health-giving benefits of your beverage.

4. How to NOT prepare your tea the right way - Of course, if there is a correct way to prepare tea, there is also an incorrect way to prepare your tea. Of course, these include poor preparation techniques most people do while making their tea. Beyond preparation, this book will also tell you about the ingredients that are not advisable to be added in tea because it either negates the weight-shaving properties of tea or kills the nutritional benefits.

5. Simple healthy tea recipes - There are so many ways to prepare tea, as evidenced by the explosion of numerous tea stores all over the world. This book will teach you how to prepare café-quality tea recipes easily at home. Not only will these recipes put most store-supplied concoctions to shame, but they are also prepared in such a way that it maximizes the health benefits you can get from tea.

Those are just some of the things you can learn from this book. My aim is that by the end of this book, you are able to prepare tea like a boss and lose that excess weight in the process. Get in the best shape of your life with the help of tea!

The Health and Weight Loss Benefits of Tea

"Tea is very healing."

- Kristin Chenoweth

Tea is one of the healthiest drinks you can ever get for yourself. This has been proven often over the years. Our ancestors drank it to keep their body running efficiently. At the same time, modern research has shown that there are scientific facts to match these seemingly lofty claims. From ridding one's body of toxins to shedding off excess pounds, regularly drinking tea greatly helps in keeping you healthy, regardless of your age. This chapter will let you take a look on how regularly drinking tea can improve the state of your health and reduce your weight at the same time.

Numerous health benefits are associated with constant consumption of tea. It does not really matter what kind of tea you prefer consuming. As long as it is of the natural kind (and as long as your drink contains the right ingredients), tea can give a boost to your health in a variety of ways. The following are just some of them.

1. Detoxification - Removing the toxins from your body is very important. When left unchecked, toxins left inside your body can cause various health problems such as cancers. While other people go to great lengths to rid their bodies of toxins, one of the easiest ways to do it is by drinking tea with regularity. Tea is an amazing source of antioxidants that help in eliminating free radicals. At the same time, tea can stimulate proper bowel movement, which helps in reducing waste materials from digestion.

2. Prevention of aging-People are looking for all kinds of ways to stave off aging. Drinking tea was clinically proven to protect your body from aging both inside and out. Tea naturally contains antioxidants such as polyphenols that help in eliminating free radicals. By removing free radicals, it is possible to prevent cell

destruction. At the same time, studies show that tea helps in strengthening elastin and collagen, 2 proteins naturally found in skin, bones and cartilage. This effect prevents joint erosion and the development of wrinkles.

3. Stress relief - Relieving stress is one of the keys for holistic health. Tea is one of nature's best stress busters. It is one thing that drinking tea is a welcome treat after a hard day's work. It is another thing that tea is clinically proven to be a cure for stress. A study has shown that the consumption of tea lowers the levels of stress hormones such as cortisol. Also related to this, tea also lowers blood pressure, a common effect associated with stress and is a major stressor in itself. If you feel stressed out, having a cup or two of tea should be a good idea.

4. Other health benefits - There are other health benefits of tea that has been confirmed by scientific studies or at least currently under serious investigation. Tea is seen to have a positive effect on cardiovascular health as it reduces blood pressure and it is seen to improve the function of the endothelium (the inner layer of blood vessels). At the same time, it might also have a positive effect in reducing a patient's overall risk for developing diabetes. In addition, a study uncovered that it has a protective effect on the retina, which is crucial for maintaining correct eyesight.

Due to the purposes of this book, I have decided to create a completely different topic focused on how tea causes weight loss. It is a fact that drinking tea facilitates weight loss. The surprising fact is that weight loss is accomplished through multiple mechanisms. Each of these ways is beneficial in its own right. Together, these mechanisms make tea such a potent weight-busting drink. Here is the list of the different ways on how tea helps you lose weight.

1. Tea increases metabolism - Increasing one's metabolic rate is one of the keys to losing weight. The basic rule is that the higher one's metabolism is, the less likely excess calories would be transformed into fat. On the same note, an elevated metabolism causes your body to tap into your fat stores for energy, burning them off on the process. Compounds naturally found in tea such as caffeine and epigallocatechin gallate (EGCG) boost metabolism, helping you burn off food and excess fat at a higher rate. In reality, an increased

metabolism helps people lose weight, even without the help of exercise!

2. Tea helps in mobilizing stored fat - Most people find it difficult to trigger their bodies to use up their excess fat. Drinking tea can significantly help in that regard. Aside from increasing your metabolism, tea also helps in mobilizing fat by triggering changes in your hormonal levels. EGCG inhibits an enzyme that causes the breakdown of epinephrine. By increasing the body's epinephrine levels, body signals to break down fat are emphasized, causing the mobilization of fat bound inside fat cells for metabolic purposes.

3. Tea helps in increasing fat burn - Have you observed that tea or some components of tea are usually included as an ingredient for weight loss mixes? It has been backed by scientific studies that tea helps in burning fat through a combination of multiple processes. Studies show that those who drink tea burn more fats compared to those who do not. The results become more marked when the person exercises. Briefly, drinking tea combined with exercise will help you achieve significant fat loss.

4. Tea reduces appetite - As much as calorie burning is a critical part of losing weight, calorie uptake is just as crucial in determining final weight loss. One thing that can significantly help in losing weight is to reduce one's appetite and calorie intake. In numerous studies, it has been observed that calorie intake is reduced in tea drinkers. While further studies must still be done, some studies show evidence that drinking tea may help in appetite regulation. In some animal studies, it is suggested that tea consumption may reduce the amount of fat absorbed from food.

Tea can induce weight loss through multiple ways. One way of evaluating the potency of something is to see how far-reaching its effects are on the subject. If this is the basis, it is safe to assume that tea is one of the best weight loss interventions out there today. Fully natural, highly effective, loaded with positive health effects and with no harmful side effects, it is easy to see why people from all backgrounds are drinking their tea for improved health.

Tea is linked to all kinds of health benefits, with one of the most notable ones in the field of weight loss. By increasing metabolism and potentially inhibiting calorie uptake, it has been proven in numerous studies that tea has a positive effect on weight loss.

Getting to Know the Different Kinds of Tea

"We were in Japan once where they had 30 types of green tea. I thought there was one."

- Billy Corgan

Tea (except those derived from other plants such as peppermint) is usually derived from leaves of the plant Camellia sinensis. While the tea plant is considered native in China, India, and other parts of Asia, it will not be long until the plant will make it around the world. As there are different kinds of tea on the market, it will be interesting to know what the differences between these variants are. Unless specified, all the teas mentioned here are in reality derived from the same tea plant. It is more of the way the leaves are genuinely prepared that creates the different distinctions between these different types of tea.

Without bothering you so much with this introduction, here are some of the most popular kinds of tea you can find in the market today.

1. White tea - This tea is the purest of all teas. In contrast to the other types, white tea is virtually unprocessed, with the leaves not being subjected to curing or fermentation. To prepare this type of tea, the leaves are simply steamed and then dried. White tea contains only 1-2% caffeine and is distinguished by its light color and flavor. Its mild and delicate taste made it the choice of royalty in Ancient China. As for health benefits, white tea stands out as it is the most potent tea variant for its anticancer properties.

2. Green tea - This tea is considered as the most popular of them all. This is mainly because of its popularity in Asia. Compared to white tea, green tea leaves are heat-treated to prevent the fermentation of the leaves. Heat treatment is usually done by either roasting or steaming the leaves. After heating, the leaves are rolled and are allowed to dry. Green tea is named as such because they produce a

greenish drink once steeped. It has numerous unique health-giving properties. It has the highest EGCG content among all tea variants and is directly linked to preventing diseases such as cancers and hypertension.

3. Black tea - This tea, while not as popular as its white and green variants, are also being consumed in relatively high amounts around the world. Black tea gained its characteristics through a fermentation process. After fermenting the leaves, they are heated to produce the characteristic black color. This type of tea is mainly characterized by its dark color, strong taste and relatively high caffeine content. Black tea is popular in the medical community because of its caffeine content and its ability to reduce stroke and lung damage risk.

4. Oolong tea   This type of tea is becoming very popular with the masses these days. Commonly served in Chinese restaurants, this tea is popular for having a full-bodied flavor and distinctive aroma. The preparation of Oolong tea is essentially similar to that of green tea, with some additional steps. After picking the leaves, you need to shake them to induce "bruising", which initiates fermentation and oxidation. The leaves are then roasted or steamed after they have slightly fermented. This form of tea is mainly noted for its ability to lower blood cholesterol levels and potentially stimulate weight loss.

5. Herbal tea - They are not considered true teas as the leaves used for them are not derived from the tea plant. However, they are fast becoming popular for different reasons. Not only do they bring different flavors into the table, but they can also have unique health-giving properties, depending on the plant where they are derived from. They are usually very versatile to prepare and are becoming widely accepted by the tea-loving community.

More kinds of tea are out there, but these five are the most basic of them all. There are also sub-variants for each type of tea, but that is something you will learn in good time once you are fully into the tea drinking lifestyle. For now, this basic knowledge will serve you well the next time you shop for tea. It will also give you an idea on what to expect once you start drinking and comparing each tea type.

There are different kinds of tea out there. Except for herbal teas, they are all derived from the same tea plant (Camellia sinensis). The way they are prepared mainly sets the differences between each tea type.

How to Make Tea

"I think tea is more zen-like. It requires a different environment."

- Howard Schultz

In many ways, tea is just like its popular counterpart, coffee. Sure, the finished product is much predicated to the quality of the tea leaves themselves, but it also boils down to execution. How one makes his or her tea has a huge say on the quality of the finished product. Do it the right way and you are bound to enjoy a tea of absolutely high quality. Do it wrong and you'll get a drink that is unpleasant tasting and robbed of all its natural goodness. For your benefit, I decided that you must also learn the nuances of preparing tea the right way. A separate chapter will be dedicated to discussing where people go wrong. What this chapter aims to do is to help you learn the basics of preparing the perfect tea.

1. The water is very important - Water is of central importance in determining the quality of tea. Using the right water enhances the final product in many ways. Go for water that is filtered but not distilled, as distillation makes the water somewhat un-ideal for steeping. You can use tap water, but it is advisable to cool it down for at least 10 seconds before using it for tea.

2. The vessel is of equal importance-You might be wondering why the most hardcore of tea enthusiasts pay close attention to the utensils. This is because it is very important as well. It is important that the material you use for a tea pot/kettle is non-reactive. Ceramic or glass should be perfect for this purpose. You can preheat the vessel to prevent excess heat loss (more on this later) by adding a little hot water on the vessel where you will steep the tea.

3. How much tea should I use? - This is an important question most newbies ask when preparing tea. For starters, they usually go for teabags as they are usually proportioned already for a single cup. However, should you go for fresh leaves, the equation becomes a little trickier. It all depends on the type of strength of the tea leaves

themselves. To play safe, use one heaped teaspoon of tea leaves per cup. You can master proportions as you become more familiar with your tea. Just remember that not all teas are made equal.

4. Temperature is critical - On most hot drinks, all you need is to bring the water to a boil, dump the mix, dissolve, and you're good to go. This does not hold true with tea. To get the most out of your tea, you need to steep it at a very specific temperature. For white and green tea, the magic temperature is in between 75 to 85 degrees C, which is just under boiling point. For black and oolong tea, it is at 90 to 100 degrees C, which is at boiling point. As a rule of thumb, fermented tea leaves must be subjected to higher water temperatures. The right temperature ensures efficient steeping and prevents the degradation of compounds.

5. Steeping-The process of steeping entails the infusion of the contents of tea leaves into the water. Many factors dictate this process. One of them, temperature, was already mentioned earlier. The other important factor for steeping would be time. Different types of tea require different steeping times to infuse all of the contents. As a rule of thumb, the more fermented the leaves are, the longer steeping time it requires. Also, whole leaves require longer steeping than broken leaves. Never steep leaves for too long or else it would result to a bitter blend.

6. Serving - You can serve your tea either hot or cold. Make sure to remove the leaves before serving to prevent over-steeping and to prevent ingestion of leaves. If you want it hot, we recommend that you serve it immediately after steeping. If you want it cold, you can let it cool down first, place it on the fridge, or add some ice. If you will not consume the tea immediately, you can have it chilled to prevent it from going stale. You can also add some condiments or toppings on your tea to add some flavor in it.

In essence, that is the fundamental steps on how to prepare tea the right way. Get all these right, and you will have superb tea you can drink all day. You will also be able to make the type of tea you will be proud to serve to your friends.

Making tea the right way is essential to get the most out of your drink. It requires attention to detail, but the steps are really very simple. The preparation method is reasonably constant, but the time you will spend in one step depends on the type of tea you're preparing.

How to Not Make Tea

"Brewing a good cup is something not everyone can do, and I loathe bad tea."

- Rod Stewart

If there is a correct way in preparing tea, of course there would be an incorrect way of doing it! These incorrect steps will not just detract the quality of your tea, but it will also hinder its ability to help you lose weight. The degree in which weight loss is compromised is varied, but it is safe to say that to get the most of your tea, you must follow all these steps. Apart from wrong tea preparation, this chapter also contains some tea-drinking habits you must avoid from this point forward.

1. Beware of diet teas - There used to be a time when there is a so-called diet tea craze. All people must do to lose weight is to drink them and they will instantly start losing weight. However, it is crucial to note that consuming them without moderation can lead to health problems. Many of these teas contain fat blockers, laxatives, and other ingredients that would make you lose weight at the fastest possible way. Potential side effects include nausea, dehydration, diarrhea and even malnutrition.

2. Avoid tea with added sugar or sweeteners - The reason behind this logic is very simple. Sugar = calories. Extra calories are something you do not want if you are serious about your weight loss goals. If you are in the hunt for teabags (as they are convenient and beginner-friendly), check the label to ensure they are unsweetened. Natural sugar adds extra calories and can make you prone to diabetes. Artificial sugar has some potentially dangerous side effects. If you will be making your own tea, avoid adding sweeteners. You will eventually get used to it.

3. Not making tea drinking a habit - Some people think that drinking tea would yield instant results. Remember that these drinks are not intended to be a get-thin-quickly formula, and it

never was one. To get the most out of tea's health-giving benefits, it would be great to make it a habit. Make an effort to consume at least one glass of tea a day. You can prepare one while making your breakfast. You can even pack a glass of tea as you go outside.

4. Never use milk for your tea - It has been scientifically proven that adding milk to your tea is counterproductive. While the milk tea craze is sweeping the world, it is actually not the healthiest combination in the world. It has been found that casein, the protein found in milk, creates complexes with the flavonoids found in tea. This renders the flavonoids useless, negating much of the health value of tea. What's more, milk also adds calories you do not need when you are trying to lose excess weight. So yes, avoid the milk tea.

5. Not combining tea drinking with other healthy habits – Some people wrongly think that as long as they're doing something healthy at the moment, it would compensate all other bad habits they have. This deserves extra emphasis as you try a tea-drinking lifestyle. The benefits you can get from regular tea drinking would be useless if you do not embrace a healthy lifestyle. If you do not have a regular exercise regimen and you continue eating an unbalanced diet filled with excess, you will never get to your ideal weight. Combine regular tea drinking with other health benefits, and you will maximize your weight loss.

You must develop the correct habits when drinking tea. Apart from making tea drinking a habit, what you include in it has a huge say in its ultimate nutritional value. Last, but not least, do not forget that it takes more than just drinking tea to lose weight.

Some Tea Recipes You Can Do At Home

"I take my teabags with me wherever I go."

- Helen Mirren

The rising popularity of tea has resulted to the creation of all kinds of tea recipes. From teahouses to coffee shops and everywhere else in between, it seems like everyone has his or her own version of creating the ideal tea beverage. For the purposes of this book, I have placed the focus on creating tea recipes that would help you accomplish weight loss. While it has been mentioned that drinking tea pure and unadulterated is still the best way to go, getting creative occasionally should help you appreciate tea more. Here are some great tea recipes for weight loss you can prepare at home.

1. Lemon Ginger Cooler

With your experience with iced tea, you just know that lemon and tea simply works very well together. The addition of ginger in the mix not only gives a new dimension to the flavor of this drink, but it also adds a distinctive flavor too. Complementing the fat-shredding powers of tea is the ability of ginger to trigger weight loss. Ginger root helps in burning fat and reduces the reproduction rate of adipose cells.

Servings: Good for 2

Ingredients: 4 teaspoons White or Black tea, lemon grass, lemon peel, ginger root

Directions: Steep all ingredients in hot water. Ideally, the temperature must be at 195 degrees F. The drink should be ready in 3 to 5 minutes. Serve hot.

2. Spiced Green Tea Smoothie

Do you want to add some spice to your tea? This recipe can add spice to your drink, literally. The heat coming from the spices is the perfect contrast to the cool presented by the tea and ice. To sweeten the pot, each serving has less than 100 calories and it is loaded with a ton of metabolism boosting goodness. We can bet tea smoothies are not made like this in your local coffee shop.

Servings: Good for 2

Ingredients: ¾ cup prepared green tea, 2 tablespoons lemon juice, ¼ teaspoon cayenne pepper, 1 piece pear (chopped), 2 tablespoons fat-free yogurt, 2 teaspoons agave nectar, ice

Directions: Mix all ingredients inside a blender. Pulse until mixture becomes smooth. Drink while it is cold.

3. Green Tea Tonic

This is a recipe inspired by a popular Dr. Oz tea recipe called the Tangerine Weight-Orade. This remarkably simple recipe is one of the best slimming tea recipes you can find out there. It combines 2 weight-busting ingredients: green tea and tangerine. This green tea tonic is great for the summer days as it is cool and refreshing. Shredding off extra pounds while chilling out: who wouldn't want that, right?

Servings: Good for 8

Ingredients: 8 cups (2 liters) green tea, 1 tangerine or orange (sliced), 1 handful of mint leaves

Directions: While brewing the tea, mix in the tangerine so it infuses together with the tea. Cool down the mixture for around 5 minutes and then add the mint leaves. Refrigerate overnight before serving.

4. Green tea elixir

The degree of difficulty in preparing this tea is significantly higher compared to the other drinks included in this list. This drink will demand you to prepare well in advance, but I swear you are going to love the result once it is all complete. Provided you do not add any sugar or sweetener, this drink should help you a lot as you try to lose weight. It's refreshing taste and fat-burning characteristics will keep you coming back for more.

Servings: Good for 8

Ingredients: ¼ cup green tea leaves, ¼ cup lemon juice, 1 cup ginger syrup (more on this later), ¼ cup pomegranate molasses, mint leaves, lemon slices for garnish

Directions (for ginger syrup): Mix ¼ cup water and ½ cup sugar together in a saucepan. Whisk this mixture together as the syrup comes to a boil. Stir in 2 tablespoons of shredded ginger. Cool the mixture down then refrigerate overnight.

Directions (for tea): Heat 2 ½ liters of water up to 170 degrees F. Turn off heat then place tea in water. Let the tea leaves steep in the water for 5 minutes. Strain mixture and discard the leaves. Stir ginger syrup, lemon juice, and pomegranate molasses. Add 6 cups of cold water and stir. Let the mixture chill overnight. Serve over ice and garnish with lemon slices and mint leaves.

5. Lavender white tea

White tea is highly notable for its smooth taste. Combine this with the equally smooth taste of lavender and you get a drink that is fit for warm summer days. This drink is very simple to prepare and would help you lose weight in no time. To sweeten the pot, getting lavender for your drink is not as hard as you think.

Servings: Good for 4

Ingredients: 4 bags or 4 tablespoons white tea leaves, 2 teaspoons fresh lavender blossoms, sprigs of lavender for garnishing

Directions: Simmer 2 cups of water in a saucepan. Once it boils, turn off the heat and add both tea leaves and lavender. Steep for 5 minutes and then strain the mixture. Let the prepared tea cool down. Pour mixture on glasses filled with ice. Garnish with lavender sprigs if desired.

6. Green tea cranberry spritzer

This is the type of drink you will be more than comfortable to share with your friends during parties. Compared to other spritzers, this one is completely healthy and can help you lose some pounds to boot! I would bet that your folks would not even recognize that it is a full-fledged "diet drink" and made using fresh green tea! If you want to impress on your next party, then you should definitely add this mix on the menu.

Servings: Good for 4

Ingredients: 4 tablespoons fresh green tea leaves or 4 bags green tea leaves, ½ cup cranberry juice, 2 cups soda water, 1/3 cup sugar (optional)

Directions: Steep tea in 2 cups of hot water for 2 to 5 minutes. Heat 1/3 cup water in a saucepan and let the sugar completely dissolve in it. Mix together tea, sugar mixture, and cranberry juice. Distribute mixture into 4 glasses and then fill them up with soda water.

7. Green tea, kiwi, and mango smoothie

Everybody loves his or her smoothies. Something that is used to be a staple only at the tropics, it is fast becoming a favorite for people all over the world. This fruity smoothie loaded with green tea can give you all the sweetness you need (without the excess) and more. It has an abundance of vitamins as well as antioxidants and compounds that aid with weight loss and digestive health. If you are aiming to lose weight for health, do it with style by having a glass of this lovely smoothie.

Servings: Good for 4

Ingredients: 2 yellow mangoes (frozen and diced), 3 ripe kiwis (quartered), ¼ cup honey, ¾ cup unsweetened yogurt, ½ cup baby spinach, 2 tablespoons green tea, 2 tablespoons water, 2 cups ice cubes, ½ teaspoon lime rind

Directions: In a blender, place mango, half of the yogurt and honey, lime rind, and water. Process the mixture while stirring it occasionally. Place this mixture on glasses and store them in the freezer. Meanwhile, place the remaining yogurt and honey, kiwi, spinach, green tea, and ice on the blender. Once blended, place this mixture on the glasses filled with the mango mixture. Serve immediately.

8. Blueberry and tea smoothie

How about this for a detox drink? Blueberries and tea are both extremely rich with antioxidants that keep cells functioning youthfully. What's more, these antioxidants also have a preventive function against diseases such as cancer. This smoothie will not just help you get all the antioxidants you will need, but it would also help in increasing metabolism for weight loss. Furthermore did we mention that it's an extremely yummy drink too?

Servings: Good for 4

Ingredients: 2 cups fresh blueberries (frozen), 2 cups white tea (chilled), 1 cup fat-free yogurt, 2 tablespoons almonds, 2 tablespoons flaxseed, ice

Directions: Mix all ingredients together in a blender and process until smooth.

All kinds of tea recipes are out there and each one can help you achieve weight loss. Those are just some samples. Feel free to create your own mixes, provided you do not include the bad stuff in there. Good luck and have fun!

How to Apply What You've Learned?

Drinking tea is one of the best decisions you will ever make when it comes to your own health. Beyond losing weight, tea drinking as a habit can help in making your body stronger. Losing those excess pounds will be very beneficial for your health in so many ways, but the impact of tea in your health goes beyond that. It protects your cells, keeps your digestive tract running in high gear, and improves your immunity too.

Proper preparation of tea is important so you can get the most out of it. It all starts with the selection of tea. While all kinds of tea are good and of equal value, each has specific requirements, so you can get the best out of them. From water temperature to steeping time, all these factors are critical to make the best tea possible. It may take time to get used to, but trust me, all these are very important.

Apart from proper preparation, it is important to consider what you would add to your drink. While it takes some time to get used to it, I recommend that you drink your tea in its pure form. This maximizes the weight loss potential of tea and keeps calorie consumption at a minimum. If you shall add some toppings, I advise that you stick with healthy ones such as fruit and spice. Some ingredients such as sugar and milk are not recommended as these nullify many of the weight-shaving properties of tea. There are numerous healthy tea recipes out there. Feel free to research and experiment.

Last but definitely not the least, I would recommend that you combine tea drinking with other healthy habits. Get enough exercise. Eat a balanced diet. Take control of your daily habits so that your body would be in the best shape. A little discipline and a well-rounded lifestyle can go a long way in accomplishing your fitness goals.

How To Lose Weight Without Working Out

A lot of people want to lose weight but rarely have the time for routine exercises or a well-planned healthy diet. However, it's NOT TRUE that you have to control your life with military precision in order to lose weight. The fact is that weight gain happens due to the accumulation of small, seemingly inconsequential habits that we have in our daily lives.

This book is meant to help you unlearn those bad habits while learning the small, inconsequential yet *helpful* ones that can result to weight loss. By the end of this book, you will become aware of your small weight-gain habits, discard them, and replace them with small, effortless weight-loss habits.

The best part about this book is that you'd be able to shed the pounds without going through extensive and rigorous workouts or incredibly difficult diets. In fact, you won't even feel a thing – except your skinny jeans as it becomes looser and looser on your hips!

Read on and find out exactly how this book can make this happen!

You're Not Hungry

"Appetite has really become an artificla and abnormal thing, having taken the place of true hunger, which alone is natural. The one is a sign of bondage but the other, of freedom"

- Paul Brunton, The Notebooks of Paul Brunton

In the old days, people ate when they needed to – the scarcity of food didn't leave much for indulgence. Nowadays however, food is everywhere and unfortunately, it is the most commonly used stress-reliever for most people. Feeling sad? Eat! Feeling bored? Eat! Most people aren't even aware of the extent of their eating habits, believing that they're eating properly but not really counting those extra bits of chocolate they snuck in when no one's looking.

That's why the first step for weight loss without working out is simple: control your diet, starting with the sheer amount of the things you eat.

Signs You're Not Really Hungry

The problem with the body is that it can fool you into thinking you're hungry when in truth; you actually need to fill a specific need. This is why before you open the fridge thinking to satisfy your hunger, it's best to take a step back and ask yourself first: am I really hungry? Here are some signs that your stomach is really fake-growling.

Specific Food Request

A first and common sign of fake-hunger is the specificity of your food request. Real hunger doesn't identify between different food types – as long as it's edible, you will eat it – if you're really hungry. If you happen to be imagining a perfectly glazed doughnut however

26

while ignoring the fruits and vegetables in the fridge, chances are your stomach is just faking it.

Stomach Not Growling

A growling stomach is probably the strongest indicator of hunger. Once you hear sounds emanating from it, you'll know that it's been a long time since you last ate. Of course, it's not usually a good idea to wait until your stomach is making some noise before eating, but paying close attention to what your stomach *feels* like (empty, full, heavy, bloated) should give you a good idea on the status of your hunger pangs.

Instantaneous Hunger

Hunger is not instantaneous. You can't be full one moment and hungry the next, rather, the need for food should creep up on your as the body slowly uses up the food you've previously eaten.

Clock Says Otherwise

If you just ate 15 minutes ago, there's no way you can be hungry again. Typically, the human body experiences hunger in the morning, noon, and night time, hence: breakfast, lunch, and dinner. Some small hunger pangs may be felt around 9AM and 3PM – upon which you'd probably take a snack break. If you're seeking food at any time other than those mentioned, your body is just fooling you into thinking its hungry.

Still with Energy

Hunger usually leads to physical and emotional weakness. You'll find yourself becoming irritable and having a hard time moving around. Of course, it's important to note that this may not always be a sign of hunger. People who are on a high fat and sugar diet often feel sluggish or "heavy" due to the imbalance of their dietary consumption. It's best if you can distinguish between lethargy from a bad diet versus hunger weakness. If not, a low energy might bear less weight as a sign of hunger.

If even just two of these signs are present, it's best to walk away from the fridge right now! This is not actual hunger but rather, your mind fooling you into thinking you need more food. Now the question is, what do you do to distract yourself from giving in to the temptation? The next Chapter should help.

*Create a daily eating schedule. Eat only during those specific times of day.

How to Kill Fake Hunger

"Remember, you are not a heavy person trying to slim down. You are a trim, health person learning how to reemerge."

- Celso Cukierkorn

After discussing the existence "Fake Hunger", the next question would be – how do you kill this problem? Even if you *know* that you're not really hungry, the pangs are still there – which means that eventually, you'll find yourself giving in. Don't! There are ways to successfully stamp down the feeling and "fool" your body into thinking you've eaten. Here are some tips on how to do this:

Drink a Glass of Water

In some cases, "thirsty" and "hungry" become intertwined in the brain, making people think that they need food when all they really need is a tall glass of water. Therefore, when you start feeling those hunger pangs – go straight to the kitchen and pour some water down your throat. Wait at least 5 minutes...are you still hungry? Guzzle another glass and wait for 5 more minutes. If you're still feeling the same hunger then this is your "go" signal to actually eat something. More often than not however, the hunger pangs stop right there. The beauty of this technique is that for really hungry people, drinking a glass of water can actually make their stomach grumble, a sure sign of hunger. For those who aren't hungry, this helps fill the stomach and ensures that if they *do* eat, they'll consume fewer amounts of food.

Wait 15 Minutes

In most cases, 15 minutes is all it takes for your body to "forget" the hunger. This is because fake hunger is often instantaneous yet temporary. One minute, you have this very powerful urge to eat a donut and after 15 minutes or so, you won't even remember wanting a donut so badly.

Distract Yourself against Boredom

This works well with the 15-minute wait, allowing you to pass the time without watching the clock. Distraction can be in many forms, depending on what would hold your interest the longest. In most cases, simply refocusing the brain's attention is enough to stop your stomach from feeling fake hunger. Studies show that in most cases where people overeat, they are usually driven to it because they have nothing else to do, hence the frequent trips to the fridge to see what's available. It helps if you keep your day occupied with tasks or chores, therefore leaving no room for boredom.

Fighting Stress

It is often said that food is the most abused anxiety drug – which is why people who are often under a lot of stress find themselves eating every few minutes. For most, the taste and feel of food is a source of comfort, regardless of whether they feel full or not. This is often coupled with inactivity since a depressed spirit rarely wants to move. Obviously, the end result is rapid weight gain. So what do you do if stress is your main problem?

Exercise is the most underutilized anti-depressant, but that doesn't mean you have to instantly go out for a jog. Remember, we're trying to lose weight without workouts –so a different alternative to stress might become necessary. Following are some of the 'anti stress' techniques you can try out that don't involve eating or excessive physical activity:

Drink Tea

Chamomile tea is one of the most effective ways for you to relax. If this isn't to your liking, almost any other type of tea would do particularly lemon and green tea. Prepare them whenever you feel yourself becoming stressed.

Massage and Acupuncture

Individually, massage and acupuncture can offer stress relief as it targets specific areas of the body that are "locked" or experiencing tension. At least one of these every week should ensure that you end your working days relaxed with no massive appetite to deal with.

Sleep

Sometimes, the best way to handle nagging cravings and stress at the same time would be to sleep. Most people who use this technique find that when they wake up, their cravings tend to disappear. Not only that, but did you know that sleeping actually burns off more calories than watching TV?

Of course, those are just few of the techniques you can use to fight stress. It really depends on what works for you so make sure to check out different methods until you find the one you want.

*Bring a container of water with you wherever you go and take a sip whenever you experience cravings.

Easy Dietary Changes for Weight Loss

"Food is an important part of a balanced diet"

- Fran Lebowitz

Knowing how to kill fake hunger often won't cut it if you're looking to shed pounds quickly in a healthy way. It's important that you also take the time to create and follow a balanced diet to ensure that your body is getting all the nutrients it needs to stay strong. Unless you eat fast food for breakfast, lunch, and dinner however – a complete revamp of your daily diet might not be necessary. More often than not, simple dietary changes are the only things you'll have to do in order to lose weight. The great thing about these small 'steps' is that they're so simple, making them practically effortless to follow. That being said, following are the small techniques you can try out.

Warm Water in the Morning

Drink a glass of warm water in the morning before taking anything else. Two glasses of water would be best, but you can start with just one glass until you're used to the sensation. Doing so on an empty stomach helps with the digestion and ads up to your daily quota of 8 glasses. You'll find that after drinking, your stomach will grumble and you might find a need to go to the toilet – which is actually a good thing. Wait 30 to 60 minutes before eating or drinking your coffee. Some individuals also like to add a few slices of lemon into the mix, or perhaps a few teaspoons of freshly squeezed lemon juice. This has been proven to help speed up metabolism.

Water before Eating

If you're going to settle down for a meal, it's a good idea to drink a glass of water first. This not only helps the digestion but partially fills your stomach so that you won't eat as much. Taking sips every few bites also helps tremendously in keeping your appetite in check.

Make Your Veggies Easy

The main reason why people eat so much junk food (aside from the fact that they taste great, of course) is the fact that they're so easy to eat. All you have to do is open a pack and start munching – so why not use the same technique for your fruits and vegetables. Apples and grapes are easy, but if you're partial to pineapples then make sure to purchase small, bite-size ones that you can put in a convenient to-go container. Baby carrots, carrot sticks, and sliced cucumbers are also perfect as snacks, providing you that 'crunchy' feeling that satisfies the stomach. Try preparing all these at night at a leisurely pace before sealing them all in an air-tight container inside the refrigerator. This way, you can just pop in a few in your mouth whenever you feel the need to chew on something.

Go Brown

White is not the natural color of most food items such as sugar. In most cases, these white food have gone through extensive processing in order to be commercial-ready, causing them to lose their natural color. Unfortunately, along with the color they also lose vital nutrients while taking in all sorts of chemicals used for the process. This is why if you want to lose weight, it's best to shift to natural and colorful food items such as green, red, orange, and brown. Their natural colors indicate that very little processing has been done, which means that most of their nutrients are still intact.

Eat Slow and Hot

This is a common problem nowadays when people only have less than 30 minutes to eat their breakfast and lunch. What happens is that they shove in spoonfuls of food in their mouth without really keeping track of how much they're eating. The problem here is that you eat food so quickly, the stomach doesn't have sufficient time to "register" that it is full. As a result, your body might have had enough to eat but your brain hasn't gotten the message yet – causing you to feel like you're still hungry. The solution – eat more slowly. By savoring your food one morsel at a time, the stomach finds it easier to register the food and signals the brain correctly when it's finally full. Studies also show that eating your food while it's hot can boost the "fullness" effect on the body – not to mention it forces you to eat slowly.

Love the Protein

Protein is a wonderful way to boost muscle growth – but it's also known to help a person feel fuller, faster. According to studies, swapping your carbohydrate diet with protein also helps with weight loss, specifically using eggs instead of say – a bagel or a donut. In the study, those who swapped their unhealthy breakfast for eggs experienced 65% more weight loss than those who didn't.

NO Diet Food

Some industries today are at their peak because they market to the dieting population. Often sold as "diet food", these prepackaged products claim to be low-fat, low-calorie, and low-everything which makes them "perfect" for people who want to lose weight. Don't believe the hype – anything that comes prepackaged and can last for more than a week is instantly suspect and should not be considered "healthy". Come to think of it, avoid all types of diet supplements as well. Remember: you want to lose weight in a healthy manner.

Juice Up!

If you're not fond of munching on carrot sticks, you might like drinking carrot juice better – or perhaps a combination of several vegetable and fruits. It really doesn't matter what your juice combination happens to be: as long as it doesn't come in a can or bottle, you're good to go! The great thing about juicing is that you can keep it in the fridge for some time and it won't go bad on you, but not too long though! For example, if you really don't have the time to fix breakfast, try juicing up your favorite combination at night and just drink it up in the morning!

No Soft Drinks

Some food items can be eaten in moderation – but some of them should be avoided at all costs. Soft drinks fall under the latter category and can provide absolutely no help to your body, aside from the good taste. Carbonated drinks are full of sugar and are the number one reason why people gain weight. If you drink at least one 500ml bottle of carbonated drink a week – that's already too much. Ditch this and opt for less-sugary fares. Water is always best but if you really need something with flavor, fruit drinks would work (but not necessarily healthier). Always follow up a sugary drink with water.

Wine in Moderation

It's generally accepted that alcohol is chock full of calories and should therefore be avoided if you want to start shedding the pounds. However, this only works if you drink several glasses a day. One glass after a meal however would be perfect, boosting your metabolism plus giving you that extra 'kick' that would let you go to sleep peacefully. Opt for red wine – it might have more calories, but the metabolic boost it provides is more than worth it. Keep in mind though, this only works in moderation.

Go Salsa

The most common comment made by dieters when switching to fruits and veggies is the bland taste of the food. For the most part, that's true because you've gotten used to the flavor-enriched servings of processed food items. However, you'll find that in time, the food starts to become tasty and you'll actually appreciate the natural flavor and texture of the food. In the meantime though – go crazy on the condiments! Not mustard or mayonnaise but rather, salsa! The calorie savings when using this particular condiment is significantly better than ketchup and mayonnaise plus the taste is something you can definitely get used to! Spoon it on everything and make sure you always have a ready supply.

Slimming Coffee

Skip the Starbucks coffee or any caffeine drink with loads of sugar. Go for black coffee or something with just a small teaspoon of sugar. You'll find that this not only helps jerk you awake better, but the calorie count is also lower.

*Always have carrot sticks ready in the fridge and bring some with you at work to munch on.

Working Out Without the Work

"When people tell me they can't afford to join a gym, I tell them to go outside; the planet Earth is a gym and we're already members. Run, climb, sweat, and enjoy all the natural wonders that is available to you."

- Steve Marboli

When the word "exercise" is spoken, this usually brings forth images of men and women in tights, doing a run with earphones stuck in their ears. Or perhaps, you see people milling about in the gym, running on the treadmill and lifting weight – but is this exercise really looks like?

Exercise is defined as: an activity that requires physical effort.

This means that *any* form of physical activity can be considered an exercise – even if it's just you getting out of bed in the morning. The trick however is to maximize these 'exercises' so that they become equivalent to a gym visit while still molding perfectly with your lifestyle. So how exactly do you work out without working out? Here are some activities you can integrate in your daily routine that wouldn't feel like you're 'exercising'.

Taking the Stairs

Start by skipping the elevators and taking the stairs instead. This can get you where you want to go while providing you with excellent buns. A slow and steady climb will help but if you really want to get the heart rate going, it's best to climb up rapidly and feel the burn of your thighs and calves. The great thing about this is that you don't have to go down at the very moment – you just need to get to the office for a much needed rest. If you think you've had enough, it's always possible to take the elevator to your floor after a few flights.

Walking to Work

Walking to work is also another wonderful example of getting where you want to go without spending some of your hard-earned cash. In fact, walking helps you save on gas or at least the cost of commute. Of course, this might not always be a possibility, for example, your home might be too far away. If it's viable however, then do it! No need to do it daily – three times a week (MWF) should do nicely.

Drying Clothes the Old Fashioned Way

Nowadays, we tend to use the handy-dandy dryer to dry the clothes – which is perfect if you need to wear something quickly. For weekly laundry however, it's usually best to hang your clothes out to dry – allowing you to stand up, walk around and stretch those muscles as you pin clothes to the clothesline. It doesn't seem like much, but hanging clothes and taking them down after they're dry can burn hundreds of calories. The best part is that sun-drying is completely free with your clothes smelling fresher than ever.

Walking after a Meal

Sitting down after a meal hinders digestion, even if you manage to drink a glass of water afterwards. The solution: stand up and do some light walking after eating so that your stomach doesn't get "pinched" and it can continue working as needed. A good way of utilizing this time efficiently is by washing the dishes after a meal – after everything's been tidied up, your stomach should feel OK enough to sit down.

Sauna it Up

Saunas are wonderful ways to relax while losing all that excess fluid that's floating around your body. A lot of people have managed to lose weight through regular sauna as the heat helps with the removal of toxins in the body. Possible the best thing about saunas is the fact that they lead to better, smoother, and healthier looking skin.

Play Your Jam

Admit it – you also do an impromptu performance when your favorite song starts playing. This might seem like fun and games, but combining your favorite playlist with several household chores can actually make you more energetic, promotes physical movement and essentially gives your body a good workout while uplifting your mood. Make sure you have a playlist of some of your most favored songs and have it ready at all times.

Do What You Love

Sports can be incredible on the body but since you're having fun while doing it, it doesn't really count as a form of exercise. If there's any kind of sport you love doing – like badminton and swimming, then make a point of doing those at least twice a month! Find a badminton body or sign yourself up for the local pool for some frolicking and swimming. You'll find that sports don't just work towards weight loss but also helps develop the muscles and give you that incredibly toned body.

Housework

Housework can be a wonderful way to start shedding the pounds, a few decimal points at a time. It doesn't matter what kind of cleaning you happen to be doing: all of them works wonders. Dusting, throwing out the trash, fluffing the pillows, vacuuming the carpet, and various other forms of housework can help you work a few ounces of sweat. This might not seem like much, but totaled together – you're probably looking at more than 100 calories burned!

Now, there are lots of things that fall within the "housework" category. If you think this actually burns very little, you might be surprised! Here's a chart of specific housework's and the approximate amount of calories they burn for the average individual.

Housework	15 Minutes of Work
Sweeping floors	39
Mopping	43
Washing dishes (standing)	22
Cooking	17
Vacuuming	43
Carrying groceries	111
Child care	34

*Create a list of activities/chores that you can easily do manually without the aid of machinery or appliances. Do them.

Strengthening Your Willpower

"Enjoy losing weight. Enjoy eating healthy, delicious food. Do not wait until you reach your destination to feel good. Take as much happines and joy as you can from your weight loss journey."

- Harry Papas

The fact is that no matter how "small" these steps happen to be, you'll come to a point when your willpower wavers. You'll find yourself craving something or eating huge amounts of a particular food. This is understandable – especially if you're just starting out. Here's a step by step approach on how to deal with your craving-hunger-eat situation:

Step 1: Determine if you're feeling real hunger or not.

Step 2: If you're feeling fake hunger, utilize the techniques used to kill it.

Step 3: If you're experiencing real hunger, use the techniques offered on the chapter "Easy Dietary Changes for Weight Loss"

Step 4: If you still feel hungry or still craving food, start doing some of the suggestions offered in the chapter "Working Out Without the Work"

Step 5: If nothing still works, giving in to the craving is inevitable. However, that doesn't mean you'll have to consume as much as your stomach will allow. In this chapter, we'll talk about ways on how to boost your willpower.

Keep a Visual Reminder

A visual reminder gives you something to check out whenever you feel your willpower wavering. It can be a picture of you in your thinner years, or perhaps the picture of a model that has the kind of body you want. The important thing is that you don't sink into despair whenever you see this reminder but rather, it should inspire you into pushing forward with your goals.

Why Are You Doing This?

If you have a specific reason for attempting weight loss, always remind yourself of this reason whenever you feel yourself wavering. Are you doing this to look good for a wedding party, a reunion with friends, or do you simply want to look good when wearing a fashionable dress? It really doesn't matter what your reason happens to be – as long as it can fuel your willpower, then it will definitely help.

Keep it Small

Have both minor and major goals. One of the top reasons why people deter from their diet is because they have such big goals that their determination flags halfway through. If you're thinking to lose 50 pounds, try by targeting at least 4 pounds of weight loss every week. This way, you can measure every week and find out if you're meeting your weekly weight loss goal. Every pound lost at the end of the week throws fuel into the fire, allowing you to become more focused on the goal.

Willpower is a Muscle

Willpower is a muscle and the more you exercise it, the more capable you become of resisting temptation. This is why if you find yourself craving a generous slice of chocolate cake, don't shrug your shoulders and think: it's just for today. Every time you give in, you lose a little bit of willpower until you find yourself no longer sticking to your restrictions. Utilize will power at all times and always stop yourself before plunging in.

Of course, in the previous chapter, we've talked about giving in to the cravings once in a while so you're probably thinking – isn't this advice contradictory? How can I give in to the cravings while exercising willpower at all times? The next paragraph should tell you how.

Give In On Schedule

Simply put, give yourself a time and place to give in to these cravings. Assign a specific day indulge on sweet, high-fat food items. Typically, people choose Saturday or Sunday for this day, but this isn't always a good idea. Instead, you should opt for a weekday for your cheat day (Monday to Friday). This way, you'd consume less unhealthy food items because you'll be too busy with work. Assigning a weekend for cheating usually means you'd eat the whole day, significantly doubling your consumption. This technique works well as a sort of portion control.

Failed? Repeat!

Don't worry – people don't expect you to do this perfectly in just one go. If you've failed, then accept the mistake and move on. The important thing here is that you *don't give up.* Having a strong support system composed of friends and family also works wonderfully well and makes it easier for you to stay true to a healthier lifestyle.

*Whenever you feel your willpower being tested, take a deep breath and count to 3. Slowly let it out, this time counting backwards from 3 to 1. Repeat.

Small Things that Affect Your Weight Loss

"Weight loss is a sum of all your habits – not individual ones"

- Helen M. Ryan, 21 Days to Change Your Body

Most people are of the assumption that weight loss only covers two factors: what you eat and what you burn off during physical activity. The fact is that although this is the main *formula* to attain calorie deficiency, there are actually small habits that can significantly affect your goal. People don't really see these as related to weight loss but with careful study, you'll find that they actually fuel the fire of overconsumption and laziness. Here are the small things you'll need to avoid or practice in order to experience weight loss:

Watch the Clock

Studies have shown that erratic eating habits usually lead to faster weight gain and slower weight loss. This is because the body is confused about the exact time you're providing it with energy, causing it to become erratic with storage and calorie burns. The simplest solution here would be eating on time. You might think that postponing lunch until 3PM is no big deal as long as you get the food, but this might be the quickest way to weight gain.

Sleeping Schedule

Tiredness is often mistaken for hunger – which is why it's important that you are NEVER tired during the day. Obviously, the best way to make this happen is by getting 8 hours of sleep every 24 hours. It's been noted that people who work at nights tend to gain more weight – which can be due to the sudden change in eating-sleeping pattern. If you are one of these people, then it's important to treat your night time as if it was day time. For example, if you go to work at 8PM then you should wake up around 6PM and eat your "breakfast". Lunch would be around 12midnight and so on and so forth. Just make sure that you sleep at least 8 hours daily.

Size and Color of Your Plates

Believe it or not, the size and color of your plates actually affect your appetite in a very subconscious manner. Studies show that red and yellow enhances the appetite while blue inhibits it. Hence, if you want to go on a "subconscious" diet, it's probably time to switch your plate sets into the color blue. As for the size, large plates prompt people into filling them up which obviously leads to larger portion sizes. If you keep those plates small however, you'll find yourself unconsciously eating smaller and smaller amounts of the same food.

Menstrual Cycle

A common problem with most women is that with menstrual cycles comes the unbelievable craving for specific food items coupled with this extreme reluctance to move around. Even if you're not on a diet or exercising regularly, menstrual cycles can throw a huge crimp in your well-controlled lifestyle. A good way of battling this problem for women is by drinking green tea or black tea. This helps ease away the pain of discomfort of menstruation, removing the bloat you feel in your stomach and most importantly – it helps balance your palate so that you don't find yourself craving too much sweets.

No More TV Dinners

It's practically a routine for most people nowadays to eat in front of the television. Though it's definitely enjoyable, what you don't realize is that watching TV while eating makes it virtually impossible for you to keep track of your portion sizes. More often than not, individuals overeat when they watch television. The solution: turn off the TV and enjoy your meal the way you're supposed to. Eat only in the dining room with the entire ensemble that comes with it. Now, this might seem like too much for a single-person dinner, but you'll find that the action is actually very meditative, allowing you to become ready for dinner. By enjoying every morsel and experiencing every bite, you'd be able to eat slowly and therefore receive your brain's "I am full" signal as soon as the stomach sends the message.

One Hour after Dinner

Going to bed right after dinner is bad. Once you go to sleep, your metabolism slows down which basically means that everything you ate will likely turn into fat. Prevent this from happening by waiting at least an hour before going to bed. Two hours would actually work best but if you're tired – then go for it! Use the allotted one hour to mentally prepare yourself for sleep, taking a long shower, getting into your most comfortable pajamas, drinking tea and so on.

Your Clothes

Yes – the things you currently wear are definitely affecting your weight loss efforts. If you have lots of loose clothes, start throwing them away or perhaps putting them in a safe place in the attic. Loose clothes usually causes people to lose track of their weight loss efforts – simply because they feel comfortable in what they're wearing and feel like it's OK to still grow into these clothes. Instead, start buying tighter and tighter clothes – small enough so that you'd feel them touching your belly. Unconsciously, slowly shrinking your clothing collection prompts you into losing weight so that you'd continue to fit into them. It's like a reverse weight loss technique!

*Eat on time and only in places where you're supposed to eat.

How to Apply What You've Learned?

Diet and exercise aren't the only things that predict your weight gain and weight loss. After reading this book thoroughly, you now know that practically everything you do has an impact on your current weight. That being said, it's crucial for you to condense everything you've found out through this book into useful, actionable goals that would take you one painless step at a time to the body you've always wanted. Here are just some suggestions on how to apply what you've learned in this discussion.

Maintain a schedule for your meals and snacks.

Move more often.

Time yourself before giving in to cravings.

Take a deep breath whenever you're tempted – a clear mind helps you reaffirm that will power and make it easier for you to say "NO"

Have a mantra that you can repeat over and over again as a reminder.

Sip water continuously throughout the day.

The fact is that there are so many strategies you can utilize after reading this book to the last Chapter. As long as you understand the concept, you'll be in the position to make the small yet helpful changes that would shed the pounds one by one. Good luck!

How To Use Food As Your Fuel

The purpose of the creation of this book, "How to Use Food for Fuel," is actually very straightforward. The main reason why this book is created is to guide people on how they can use food to fuel their bodies. Humans, just like any living organism, require energy to keep their bodies running. The main way in which they can get their energy is through the food they eat. As you can infer, what a person eats has a huge say on their overall energy reserves.

This said, the first way this book can help you is by teaching you how food can help you gain energy. The human body is a remarkable system in itself, regulated by all kinds of processes to keep it running at a high level. The human body has a specialized and specifically ordered system that allows it to use different kinds of materials coming from food for energy. Knowing the different processes that transforms food into energy gives you a better understanding on how our bodies work and how diets should be done for maximum energy and nutrition.

The second way this book will help you is that it would teach you the basics of energy nutrition. There are three main energy sources for the human body. These are carbohydrates, proteins, and fats. Each of these so-called macronutrients is processed in different ways, providing energy and nourishment for the body on the process. Aside from teaching you the basic process on how these molecules are transformed into usable energy, you'll also learn which foods you can consume to get all these nutrients.

Last but not least, this book will tell you about other nutrients that are critical on the energy-production process. While they don't provide much energy in a caloric sense, some of these nutrients are important to ensure that your energetic functions are functioning like it should be. Vitamins, minerals, and even water play a huge role in sustaining the vitality of the human body, so learning where you can source these nutrients is crucial to attain maximum vitality.

Energy and the Living Organism

"What if we ban the word "healthy food" from our cooking vocabulary? I'm not talking about banning foods that are considered healthy. I'm talking about changing the way we think about food overall."

– Marcus Samuelsson

There are many characteristics that define a living organism. These defining characteristics are present in all levels of life, from single-celled bacteria that are microscopic in size to massive whales that are composed of at least a billion cells. One of these distinct characteristics all living organisms share is metabolism. The process of obtaining energy for various metabolic processes, it is the very basis why living organisms (except those who are capable of self-production of energy such as plants) are required to eat food.

How does one define metabolism? It is a series of chemical transformations that helps in sustaining life. Most of them are catalyzed by enzymes, proteins capable of triggering chemical reactions to proceed at an extremely swift rate. The role of metabolism in the body cannot be understated in both the molecular and systemic levels. The products of metabolism (most notably energy in the form of adenosine triphosphate or ATP) are used for other critical biological processes such as growth, reproduction, and reaction to stimuli. This essentially means that without metabolism, life will definitely cease.

The metabolic process can practically be summed up into two contrasting processes. Catabolic reactions break down large molecules into simpler ones. This is most commonly observed when food materials are digested to release energy and nutrients. Anabolic reactions combine smaller molecules to create bigger ones. One example of an anabolic reaction is the formation of various proteins from individual amino acids. However, one must note that catabolic and anabolic reactions usually take place simultaneously on normal states. This is one underestimated element of the magic inside living bodies.

Depending on how an organism obtains the necessary substrates for metabolism, a living being can be classified either as an autotroph or a heterotroph. An autotroph is capable of producing food from inorganic matter. Because of this, they can essentially do self-sustenance at the right physiological and environmental conditions. Examples of autotrophs include plants, photosynthetic algae/fungi, and photosynthetic bacteria. In contrast, a heterotroph cannot produce its own food. This is why they must procure it from other sources. They usually procure it from other living matter such as plants, animals, and bacteria.

This heterotrophic state is essentially the basis on why animals such as humans are required to eat food. While they have physiologic systems that help them sustain homeostatic functioning for a specific time period without food, relying on such systems is self-destructive in the long run. Eventually, there would be a time when they'll have to find a way to get food. It's as simple as that. It's why heterotrophic organisms of all levels (including humans) have developed complex structures and strategies to get food and stay nourished. Energy acquisition is an essential determinant of survival. It's simply the way of life.

The main thing you must learn in this chapter is that most organisms, including humans, are reliant in food to create energy and other vital nutrients for survival.

What You Need to Know about Food

"I like to eat and I love the diversity of food."

– David Soul

Food is an ever-splendored thing. It can mean different things to different people, and it can stand for meanings that go beyond what it really is. Food can be defined in all kinds of ways, but for the purposes of this book, we'll define food according to what it is in a scientific sense.

Strictly speaking, food is any kind of substance that can be used to provide nutritional nourishment for a living organism. Typically consisting of organic matter, food usually originates from other living material such as plants and animals. Once food is ingested by the body, it is then transformed into various components useful for an organism's survival by the process of metabolism. Energy in the form of ATP is one of the most important byproducts of metabolizing food as it drives other essential bodily functions.

The pursuit of food is one of the biggest triggers of the constant evolution of living organisms. Living things have developed all kinds of structures and strategies to ensure they'll gather enough food to sustain themselves in the everyday struggle of life. These adaptations (together with other forms of adaptation) have caused the flourishing of life and the creation of other life forms. Looking at this perspective, it is easy to say that the pursuit of food is one of the main driving forces of evolution.

The same way that food has triggered the evolution of life in general, it has also triggered the evolution of humans in particular. While humans don't have overwhelmingly powerful adaptations (ex. extreme speed, strength, and sensory acuity), they have a powerful weapon on their arsenal: the brain. The human's strong brain efficiency allowed them to adapt to just about every kind of situation and surmount most obstacles Mother Nature throws at them. In the pursuit of a long-term solution for a sustained food source, civilization as we knew it was created as a byproduct.

Historically, humans obtained their food via the hunting-gathering method. Such a lifestyle made them nomads, a lifestyle that is equal parts risky and energy-consuming. Eventually, humans have discovered that they can cultivate specific plants and animals as a source of food, giving birth to agriculture. Because the need to hunt and gather was significantly reduced, humans began establishing colonies at fixed locations. Freed from the responsibilities of looking for food, humans began to focus on other things such as social order, education, and the like. Little by little, civilization as we know it was created, and it all started when we were able to create a sustainable way to procure food through agriculture.

No matter what happens to the world, the pursuit of food will never cease. Both humans and non-humans are dependent on food to get energy and more, and this need would continue to shape the evolution of life. This awareness makes us see food in a completely different light, and on the long run that might be for the best.

Food is essential for sustaining all forms of life. Food also plays a huge role in determining the fates of all living organisms. More than just being a source of physiological sustenance, food has shaped the growth of human civilization as well.

Carbohydrate: The Primary Energy Source

"The brain needs fuel right away, and carbohydrate is the best source."

– Andrew Weil

The bodies of living organisms are made in such a way that they're able to maintain their energy levels in most situations. While almost every kind of biomolecule can be utilized to provide energy for the body, the most important energy source of them all is carbohydrates. Carbs are considered the best option for a quick, strong dose of energy, and for good reason.

Carbohydrates, as the name would suggest, are compounds that are composed of carbon, hydrogen, and oxygen. Essentially, they are hydrated carbon molecules (meaning they contain water), hence the name "carbo-hydrate". Found in either aldehyde or ketone form, individual carbohydrate molecules can combine together to form complex, biologically active molecules. Carbohydrates are the most abundant form of macromolecule found in living organisms.

The most basic form of the carbohydrate is the monosaccharide. They are usually colorless and water-soluble. At the same time, they have a crystalline structure, a derivative of its uniform molecular structure. By nature, each monosaccharide is composed of anywhere between four to seven molecules of carbon, with six molecules being the most common. These monosaccharides can also link together to create complex sugars such as disaccharides, oligosaccharides, and polysaccharides. The most biologically significant monosaccharide of all is glucose, a well-known substrate in virtually all metabolic pathways in cells. Other biologically significant monosaccharides include ribose, galactose, and fructose.

The main purpose of carbohydrates is to provide energy for living cells. Other than being metabolized to create ATP via aerobic and anaerobic processes, carbohydrates such as glucose can also be utilized for other purposes. Glucose molecules are fused together to create energy storage molecules such as glycogen in animals and amylose in plants. Carbohydrates can be used to create both lipids and proteins. Carbohydrates (ribose and deoxyribose) are also components of both DNA and RNA. They also serve a structural function in some organisms, as in the case of chitin and cellulose.

One of the main characteristic of foods rich in carbohydrates is its sweet taste. This makes carbohydrate-rich foods such as fruits a very fulfilling meal for almost all animals. That might have been an evolutionary adaptation in itself, an affirmation of the high stature of carbohydrates in an organism's health.

Carbohydrates, mainly through glucose, serve as the main energy source for practically all biological entities. Aside from being the cell's main energy source, they are also instrumental for a number of vital physiological functions.

Where to Get Your Carbs

"The more refined the carbohydrates, the greater the effect on our health, weight, and well-being."

– Andrew Weil

Carbohydrates are found in all kinds of forms. Considered as the most common form of biomolecule, you can find it in just about every kind of food. The only conflict left to be resolved would be finding the best sources to achieve optimal health. Here are some of the best carbohydrate sources you can get your hands on. As long as you consume these foods at the right amounts, not only would you have an abundance of energy to last the day, but you can also protect yourself from various kinds of diseases.

1. Fruits– Fruits and berries are one of the oldest food sources for humans. In many ways, it is still among the most effective ones you can find out there. Fruits have an abundance of natural glucose that's easily assimilated for energy production. Aside from providing a direct shot of energy, fruits and berries also contain a large amount of vitamins and minerals that are essential for keeping our normal body functions running. If you want a direct shot of energy, you can't go wrong with chomping on some fruits.

2. Whole grains– Grains are known for being stockpiles of carbohydrates. After all, they contain a high concentration of starch that is easily converted into glucose. Whole, unrefined grains are the better choice when shopping for grains such as wheat, oats, and rice. They have high levels of complex carbohydrates that are digested slowly, keeping blood glucose levels stable on the process. At the same time, whole grains have more than their fair share of dietary fiber which aids in digestive efficiency and keeps the intestines clean. Whole grain and products made out of it (ex. breads and pasta) should be included in your shopping list.

3. Energy bars– The word energy bar can be quite misleading, as most people associate it with candy bars that can be potentially

harmful in the long run. When we talk about energy bars, this refers to the ones specifically designed for such a purpose. These bars contain ingredients that are quickly assimilated by the body and yet would not cause side effects such as crashing. The best ones are made out of energy-dense natural foods such as nuts, fruit, and whole grains. They contain a massive dose of carbohydrates, just the right amount of protein, and are low in fat, ideal for providing that shot in the arm when you need it.

While carbohydrates can be found literally everywhere, selecting the right sources is very important. For sustained energy (and health preservation), it's best to go for all-natural food or those made with minimal processing. Carbs are high-octane fuel for our bodies.

Protein: An Unlikely but Effective Power Source

"Calories from protein affect your brain, your appetite control center, so you are more satiated and satisfied."

– Mark Hyman

While protein is known to perform all kinds of tasks for the human body, it is not exactly known to be a source of energy. In fact, unlike carbohydrates and fats, the body does not store protein for deployment as a reserve fuel source. Still, when the need arises, protein can be tapped as an energy source. Furthermore, protein in the form of enzymes plays a critical role in triggering all the necessary reactions for energy production. So, to say that protein is virtually useless for energy production would be both wrong and short-sighted.

The main role of protein for physiologic energetics would be its enzymatic role. Metabolism in both the cellular and systemic levels is highly reliant on enzymes to commence. For example, a glucose molecule cannot be transformed to ATP molecules without the series of enzymes that catalyze both glycolysis and Krebs cycle. Looking at the big picture, without the enzymes produced at the stomach and intestines, we cannot break down carbohydrates, protein, and fats into simpler molecules that make them easier to absorb. Needless to say, proteins in the form of enzymes play a central role in both the creation and use of fuel by all living bodies.

One of the main roles of protein in our bodies is that it's the main component of body tissues. As such, most of the proteins we obtain through our diet get channeled to the building and maintenance of tissues such as muscles. However, during extreme situations, muscles can be tapped as fuel source. When we are on a starved state, or in the middle of extreme endurance exercise, the body taps on protein found in muscles as a source of fuel. Protein can be broken down to its individual amino acids, and these amino acids can be converted into glucose. It is considered as a sacrificial system though, as it causes the breakdown of muscles.

Protein, while it represents roughly only five percent of a human being's fuel needs during normal physiologic states, plays a big role in biological energetics. In the form of enzymes, it is instrumental in converting food into usable fuel. It can also be tapped as an emergency source of glucose during times of stress. While providing fuel is not the main role of protein, it can be one when the situation calls for it.

Protein is not all that important as a source of fuel. Its main importance lies in its ability to trigger the necessary processes for converting fuel into energy. Also, it can serve as an alternative fuel source during strenuous exercise and prolonged fasting.

Where to Get Your Proteins

"I eat a variety of foods like vegetables, fruit, and beef for protein and iron."

– Sasha Cohen

We live in a relatively protein-hungry world. With more people more or less following a carnivorous diet and fitness buffs espousing the merits of a diet rich in protein, getting more of it seems out of the question. In fact, there is an argument that humans in general might be consuming too much protein these days, resulting in diseases such as gout. Still, protein is considered as a vital nutrient for a reason, so you just can't turn away from it totally. This chapter will list some of the best sources of protein you can get your hands on.

1. Lean meat– The fact that animal protein is still the best out there is inescapable. While it can be argued that full-time vegetarians can get their protein requirements without the help of meat consumption, it's actually trickier to accomplish. The main reason why animal protein is considered superior is because it comes complete with all the amino acids your body needs, including the essential ones. For those keeping score, an essential fatty acid is one that cannot be created by the body, hence the need for it to be supplemented via the diet. Go for leaner cuts of meat as much as possible. At the same time, go for relatively uncommon yet healthy animal protein options such as seafood.

2. Eggs– This has been considered as a staple meal for aspiring bodybuilders for the longest time. Of course, there's a good reason behind such a habit. The protein found in eggs is considered to be of extremely high quality as it's easily assimilated by the body. At the same time, it is considered to be nutrient-dense, boasting a high amount of protein per unit serving. It also comes with other beneficial nutrients such as minerals, healthy fats, and "good" cholesterol. Unless you are hypertensive, consuming one egg daily is considered healthy.

3. Beans– Legumes in general are great sources of plant-based protein. However, beans have a special place in the hierarchy of protein sources. Compared to other plants sources, beans are highly concentrated in protein, easily matching those found in some animal sources. Some beans even contain almost all the essential amino acids your body needs. It is estimated that the protein content found in beans approximates that of a steak of equal serving. To cap it off, beans are rich in dietary fiber, which helps in digestion and will keep you feeling full longer.

There are many ways to get protein without compromising your health in other departments. Provided that you consume them at the right amounts, animal sources are still your best source of dictary protein. Plant sources are also great alternatives as they bring unique health benefits to the table as well.

Fats: Your Power Repository

"Increase your consumption of healthful fats."

– David Perlmutter

Fats have garnered a negative rap over the past years because of their role in modern health problems such as obesity and cardiovascular disease. However, fats should never be taken out of our diet because of these reasons. Remember that fats do play a huge role in our bodies, and the diseases we get from them are diseases linked to excess. To get a better idea of why we should never shy away from fat, you must learn first its value in bodily functions.

The main role of fat in our bodies is that it serves as a repository of fuel for the body. Fat in the form of triglycerides is considered as the most concentrated form of fuel in the body. To put into perspective, each gram of fat can generate nine calories. This is a significant leap compared to carbohydrates and proteins that can generate four calories per gram each. When fat is broken down, it can provide a serious amount of energy. In fact, if all the fat stored in a typical human's body is tapped for energy, it's actually good for at least 100,000 calories!

Aside from being a highly concentrated storage form of energy, fats are also ideal storage molecules because they occupy minimal mass inside the body. Unlike glycogen, fats don't have to be stored with water, significantly cutting the potential weight and space the body would carry. At the same time, excess calories are easily converted into fat through relatively uncomplicated processes with minimal energy expenditure.

There are four main sites in the body wherein fats are available. The most common way it is stored is through adipose tissue. Found in different parts of the body such as the skin, adipose cells are specifically designed for storing fat. It can also be found in the blood in the form of free serum triglycerides. Another repository of fat would be in the muscles, immediately being tapped into once muscle glycogen becomes depleted.

Perhaps the only downside of using fat for energy is that it takes a lot of oxygen to actually decompose fat into forms that can be used as body fuel. It's actually the reason why aerobic exercise is considered the best method for burning off excess fat. Also, because of the relative difficulty of the process for using fat as fuel, it's mainly considered as an energy source secondary to carbohydrates. Still, fats are tailor-made for their purpose: as a high-powered reserve energy source.

Fats are considered as the reserve fuel source of humans and other animals. Often utilized when the body's reserve carbohydrates (free glucose + glycogen) are depleted, fat generates the highest amount of energy per unit gram among all fuel biomolecules.

Where to Get Your Fats

"Even though we're dramatic, we move our faces, we eat higher fat foods, we're the ones with fewer wrinkles. It makes you wonder."

– Salma Hayek

Now that you know that fats are not bad as long as they are not present in excess, it would be vital to also know where you can get your daily fix of fats. Not all fat sources are made equal. For example, some are abundant on carcinogenic trans fats while others are abundant in saturated fats that are potentially destructive to your cardiovascular system. Just as important as regulating your daily fat consumption, it would also be a great idea to qualify which foods you would be relying on as a fat source. This list consists of some of the best sources of healthy fats you can consume daily.

1. Fish– Certain fishes, particularly those that thrive in deep sea waters, have meats with a high amount of fat. While some dieters may pause upon hearing this, fishes such as tuna, sardines, mackerel, and salmon are among the healthiest sources of fat around. They have an abundance of omega-3 fatty acids that promote the healthy functioning of both nervous and cardiovascular systems. It also helps in reducing the effects of inflammatory diseases such as rheumatoid arthritis. What's more, fish is a great source of protein and other nutrients.

2. Avocado– This is one of the deceptively great sources of fats out there. There used to be a time when people were shying away from consuming avocados because of their egregiously high concentration of fat (a medium-sized avocado contains around 30 grams of fat!). However, more nutritionists are now recommending the consumption of avocados because most of its fat content is composed of healthy monounsaturated fats. Such fats are directly linked to lowering bad cholesterol levels in the blood. As long as it's consumed in regulation, there's no reason why you can't enjoy an avocado or two.

3. Olive oil– This is considered as one of the most premium forms of edible oil for a reason. This Mediterranean staple is considered perhaps the healthiest form of vegetable oil around. One reason why it's considered to be healthy is because of its high concentration of monounsaturated fatty acids that lower bad cholesterol levels in the blood without resorting to medications. In fact, 80 percent of this oil's fat content is of the unsaturated kind, mainly oleic acid. Olive oil is highly regarded to be cardioprotective, increasing HDL levels while reducing the risk of atherosclerosis.

It is not just about how much fat you ingest in a day, but it is also about what kinds of fat you ingest. While the fact that your daily fat consumption should always be regulated, you are best served to eat higher servings of good cholesterol and unsaturated fats.

Other Nutrients Important for Body Energetics

"It's better to get the nutrients you need from food, not supplements."

– Gail Simmons

Macronutrients such as carbohydrates, fats, and proteins can provide the raw ingredients necessary to produce energy. However, it is not enough that you have a fuel source to create energy. You also need to have other components to ensure that your energy production processes operate like they should. Just like in a machine, other additives either initiate or amplify the process of burning fuel. Here are some nutrients you must consume to keep your energy levels up.

1. Vitamin C– This vitamin, also known as ascorbic acid, is better known for its role in boosting immunity and as an antioxidant. What most people don't know about Vitamin C is that it also plays a huge role in bioenergetics. This is because it helps in maintaining the health of the adrenal glands, a crucial part of the energy production pathways in humans. Also, it helps with iron absorption (more on the role of iron later). Malaise and lethargy, two symptoms associated with the Vitamin C deficiency disease scurvy, are proof of this vitamin's role in energy production.

2. Iron– This mineral plays a massive role in ensuring that the body has enough energy to last the day. This mainly stems for iron's role in the chemical structure of hemoglobin, the protein that binds oxygen into the blood. If there is not enough iron, it results in anemia, a condition where there's either not enough red blood cells or hemoglobin. One of the presentations of anemia is general weakness because the patient experiences lack of oxygen circulation. Have enough iron in your system, get enough oxygen circulation in your system, and you'll feel significantly livelier almost right away.

3. Magnesium– This is another mineral that you must consume for increased energy reserves. The effects of magnesium in our bodies with regards to energy consumption are twofold. First, it is considered as one of the factors needed to make the cellular metabolic pathways proceed. Hence, without enough magnesium, you cannot create enough ATP. Also, magnesium is well-known for inducing rest. It aids in the relaxation of muscles and also induces sleep. All in all, magnesium fuels us by triggering our metabolism and helping us rest.

4. Potassium– This mineral is one of the best minerals for instantaneously boosting our energy. Potassium plays a very important role in muscle contraction. Once muscle cells run out of potassium, they aren't able to contract like they use to, either resulting to increased weakness or a higher propensity of cramps. Other than this, potassium also has a big role in maintaining proper water balance and a normal heart rate. Squash and bananas are among the best sources for this all-important mineral.

5. B Vitamins– All the B vitamins play a vital role in energy metabolism. While these vitamins share a common name, each is actually chemically distinct from one another. However, it was observed that most of these vitamins are found on the same foods and all play a role in converting fuel from food and storage molecules into energy. A deficiency in any of these nutrients would result to generalized weakness. There's a good reason why B vitamins are always included as an ingredient in all energy boosting products.

It is not enough that you get enough macronutrients into your system for fuel. You'll also need micronutrients such as vitamins and minerals to ensure all that fuel would be converted into usable energy.

A Sampling of the Best Energy Foods

"I like to take care of myself and know what foods I should be eating."

– Doutzen Kroes

A number of foods have already been mentioned in different parts of this book to be specifically helpful in promoting energy production. Still, I find it potentially helpful if I can include some more foods that you can add to your diet to significantly boost your energy levels. These foods, combined with healthy habits, can take your energy up another notch and make you more effective in your everyday tasks.

1. Spinach– Remember how Popeye became super powerful when he was able to eat his spinach? As it turns out, there is actual scientific basis on the secret weapon of one of the greatest characters of the cartoon world. Spinach is rich in magnesium, a nutrient that relaxes the muscles and catalyzes energy production. The combination of pumped up muscles and available energy translates to explosive muscular performance, an indicator of superior energy.

2. Banana– This is one fruit that you must not leave out from your food list. Just like most fruits, it has an abundance of glucose that translates to an instantaneous energy boost. Beyond this, it also contains vitamins that help in the body's immune function. It's also one of the best natural sources of potassium, which is vital for maintaining muscular and cellular function. A banana for dessert is great fuel for the day.

3. Melon– Melons are one of the most underrated energy-giving foods out there. Whether it's a watermelon, a honeydew, or a cantaloupe, melons are packed with a lot of energy-giving nutrients. Aside from having a good amount of vitamins and minerals per serving, they also contain a lot of water. Keeping yourself hydrated is one of the best ways to preserve your energy. In fact, studies have

shown that preventing water loss is one of the best ways to sustain energy.

4. Oats– This is one grain that stands out when it comes to providing your body with enough fuel. First, it is mainly composed of complex carbohydrates that are digested slowly. This prevents the flooding of glucose in the bloodstream (one cause of energy swings) and also ensures that there's a sustained flow of glucose in the bloodstream for longer periods, which regulates irregular hunger cycles that affect energy. Also, its abundance of dietary fiber allows for prolonged digestion, ensuring efficient breakdown and absorption of nutrients.

Food should always be your main source of fuel. Choosing the right stuff would be the first step towards ensuring peak physical performance. By including these foods in your diet, you can be assured of sustained energy throughout the day.

How to Apply Key Ideas for the Best Results?

For humans, food is and will always be the fuel for our bodies. Hence, it can be said that the food we eat would provide the fuel we need to accomplish everything that we need to do in order to strive and thrive. That said, what we need to do to ensure that our bodies would always be in peak condition is straightforward: it all starts with the food we eat. Here are some of the key ideas you must apply to get the best results.

1. Have enough carbohydrates– Carbohydrates are your primary source of energy. As they are easily transported in the bloodstream and assimilated by your cells, carbs can instantly fuel your body. Simple carbohydrates are great for an immediate energy boost, while complex carbohydrates are great for ensuring you have enough energy for the entire day. A steady mix of fruit and whole grains is all you need for a healthy dose of carbohydrates.

2. Have enough proteins– Proteins are not considered to be a primary source of fuel, but they do play a major role in keeping your energy up. First, proteins can be tapped as an emergency fuel source during times of starvation. Second, proteins in the form of enzymes play a critical role in keeping your metabolic processes running. Get your protein fix through both plant and animal sources.

3. Have enough fats– While they are maligned by many, fats do have strategic importance in bioenergetics. As the primary storage source of energy for the body, they are extremely valuable for sustaining our bodies during prolonged activity and fasting. Also, fats are the most energy-dense fuel for our bodies. As long as they are consumed in moderation, healthy fat sources are critical in maintaining a healthy body.

4. Have enough vitamins and minerals in your diet– Vitamins and minerals, while they are not directly utilized by the body as fuel, play a crucial role in ensuring vital body functions stay running. Have enough doses of them and your body will run like a well-oiled machine all the time. Both plant and animal food sources will

provide you the necessary vitamins and minerals you need. The key to getting all these nutrients is to keep your diet balanced.

5. Keep your body in shape- Beyond eating the right food for fuel, there are many ways to ensure your body will perform at the highest level. Getting enough rest and sleep would ensure that your body will recuperate from the wear and tear of daily activities. Getting enough exercise keeps your body systems in top shape. Last but not least, avoiding stress and other stressful agents would greatly help in maintaining your physical vitality.

www.ingramcontent.com/pod-product-compliance
Lightning Source LLC
Chambersburg PA
CBHW060643290526
45793CB00001B/378